The SHIIT
Workout

THE SHIIT WORKOUT

An Hachette UK Company
www.hachette.co.uk

Summersdale Publishers Ltd
Part of Octopus Publishing Group Limited
Carmelite House
50 Victoria Embankment
LONDON
EC4Y 0DZ
UK

www.summersdale.com

Printed and bound in Malta

ISBN: 978-1-78783-326-5

Substantial discounts on bulk quantities of Summersdale books are available to corporations, professional associations and other organizations. For details contact general enquiries: telephone: +44 (0) 1243 771107 or email: enquiries@summersdale.com.

The advice in this book is purely for the purpose of entertainment and should not be followed.

The SHIIT
Workout

Get Fit While You Sh*t

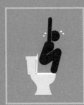

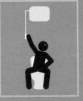

Jim Squits

summersdale

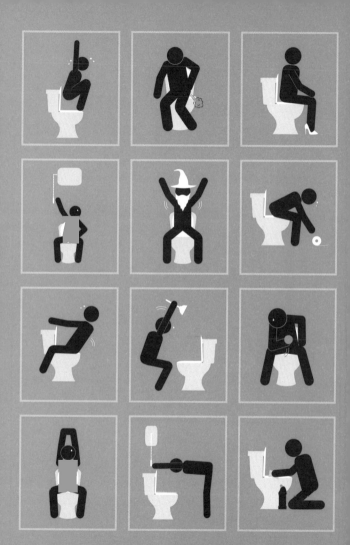

Contents

Introduction

The SHIIT workout is the smart way to get fit while you shit. Working it out has never been more fun as you go through the motions from jumping jacksies and pull-ups to shit-ups and skidders. Begin with the gentle warm-up exercises; it's important to limber up before the main event – if you SHIIT too soon, you could incur an injury as well as having a lot to clean up afterwards. Use the planner at the back of the book to log your SHIIT sessions and unload your own ideas to make SHIIT work for you. This is your essential guide to getting fit with SHIIT.*

Now, let's get ready to do some serious SHIIT!

*Beware of imitations, such as
Crap Cardio and Turd Treadmill.

It's always advisable to speak to a health practitioner before beginning a new exercise regime. In the case of the SHIIT workout, try not to stray too far from the bathroom, and make sure you have a plentiful supply of toilet tissue.

How SHIIT Works

SHIIT helps you get fitter on the shitter. With these exercises, you too can have the body of a true ass-thlete like me, Jim Squits, and a happy bowel to match. Who doesn't love a good sit down on the toilet? Well, now you can get fit as you savour those quiet moments of contemplation on the porcelain throne.

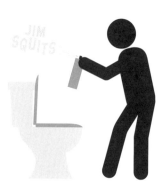

Equipment List

- A well-ventilated bathroom

- A good, old-fashioned pull
  chain for those reaches

- All-in-one Lycra, preferably
  in shades of brown

- Masses of toilet roll

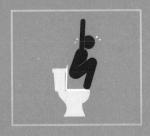
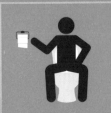
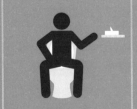

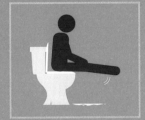
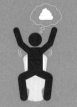
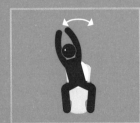
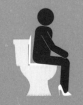

Warm-Ups

Go easy on your nether regions; don't remonstrate with your rectum or pull on that groin. Similarly, you don't want to adopt a scattergun approach to SHIIT, because that's just plain disgusting. Instead, begin with these gentle stretches to loosen up on the loo before attempting the SHIIT workout.

The Loose Bowel Lift

DIFFICULTY RATING:

This is a simple exercise to ensure correct posture for a good quality SHIIT. Squat above the toilet (standing on the seat) with knees hip-width apart and facing forwards, and keep your back straight. If you struggle with this, balance a toilet roll on your head.

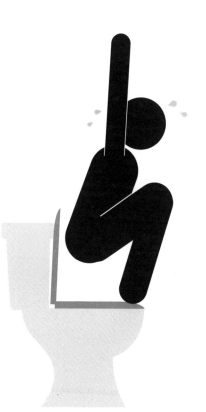

The Bog Roll Stretch

DIFFICULTY RATING:

There's nothing worse after a satisfying SHIIT than to discover that there's no bog roll and having to do an awkward sideways dance as you negotiate your way to the storage cupboard, or, worst-case scenario, call for help. This stretch helps to avoid this embarrassment as well as warming up those biceps.

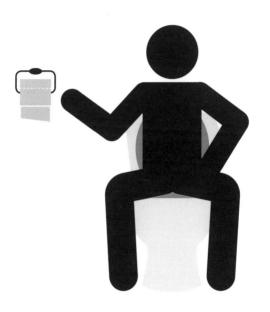

The Slider

DIFFICULTY RATING:

Some of us like to use wet wipes (fully
biodegradable and flushable, of course)
for an extra-safe wipe. For some reason
they are always in a different place to the
toilet roll, but just think of this as another
opportunity for a warm-up stretch.

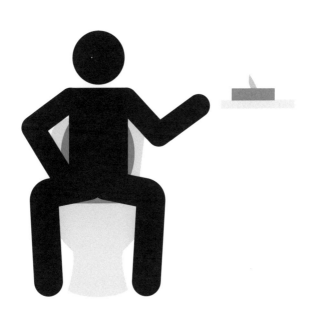

The Stench Clench

DIFFICULTY RATING:

Before busting out those toilet tunes, try to hold it in with a solid butt clench, then release to the side on a count of three.

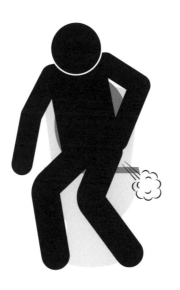

The Skidder

Let's pretend the last person to use the loo had a bad aim and the floor is somewhat slippery. Sit squarely on the toilet and skid your feet against the floor until your legs are extended. Complete five sets.

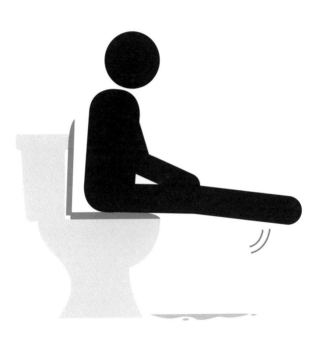

It Was This Big!

DIFFICULTY RATING:

Now imagine you are out impressing
your mates on a Friday night by regaling
the monstrous girth of the turd you
dropped earlier that day. Stretch out
your arms, with elbows bent as if holding
said monster. Feels good, doesn't it?
Hold this position for a count of ten, then
repeat five times, each time extending
the arms slightly further apart.

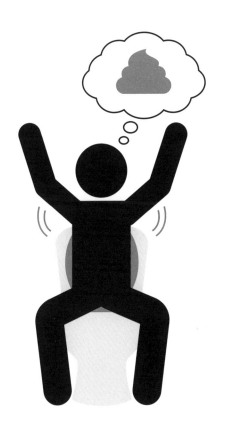

The Butt Nugget

DIFFICULTY RATING:

The gentle rocking motion of this exercise is for those occasions when your poo just won't budge. Rock on the hinge of your hips, left to right, with arms arched to frame your beautiful face. Repeat ten sets. Yeah, you're really moving now!

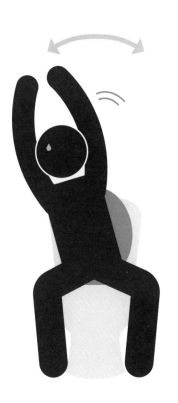

The Heel-Toe Hoedown

DIFFICULTY RATING:

They say that the best position for
a shit is to imagine you're wearing
high heels. Lift your heels and drop,
lift and drop. Repeat ten times.

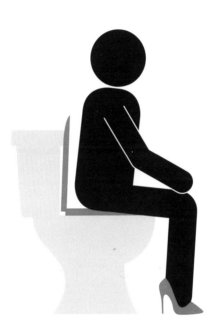

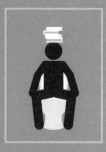
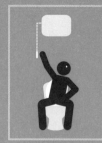
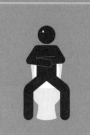
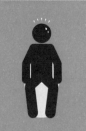
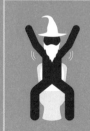
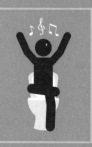
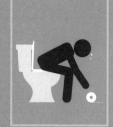
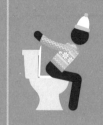
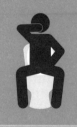

Beginner's SHIIT Exercises

Now you're loosened up and ready for
the best SHIIT of your life! Let's go!

Toilet Book Balance

DIFFICULTY RATING:

Just because you're in the smallest room doesn't mean you can ignore etiquette and decorum, and as an added bonus you'll be improving your posture. Grab a small pile of your favourite toilet books, sit up straight and balance them on your head.

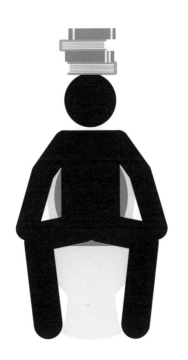

Pull-Ups

DIFFICULTY RATING:

This is where the old-fashioned pull
chain comes into its own. Stretch
up the arm nearest to the chain
and reach as high as you can. Hold
for a count of ten and release.

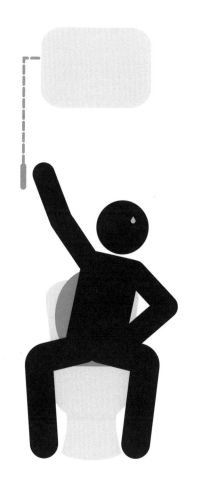

The Floater

DIFFICULTY RATING:

No, not *that* kind of floater! This requires
strong calves as you raise yourself off
the seat to a standing position, while your
arms are crossed. Repeat ten times.

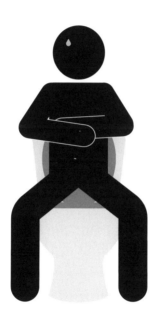

Snapshat

This one requires great care and expert bowel control. Sit squarely on the toilet as though you're preparing for a long session. Then clench your buttocks to a count of three and release to a count of three. Keep going for ten sets and try not to squeeze one out.

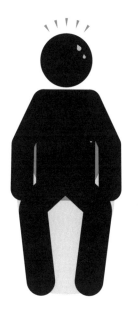

Lord of
the Ring

DIFFICULTY RATING

Malodorous hot winds from deep down
below should be stirring by now. It's
time to prepare to drop the hobbits off
at the pool. Sit up straight and stretch
those arms up high. Reach as high as
you can to the left, then to the right.
Repeat ten sets. Looking good, Gandalf!

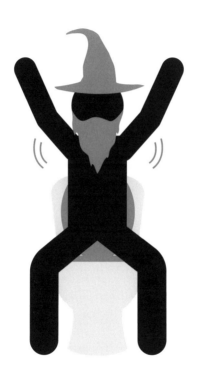

The Dingleberry Dance

DIFFICULTY RATING:

Get up and dance until the dingleberries
are ready to drop! Rise from the
seat and lift those knees!

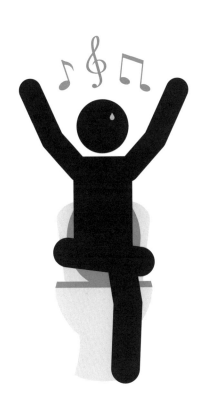

The "I Dropped the Bog Roll"

DIFFICULTY RATING:

This requires dexterity and it's also a useful move in your arse-nal when you have dropped the bog roll and haven't yet "finished". Lean forward, tummy against your legs and reach down to the floor, before doing a big scooping motion to gather the toilet roll. Phew!

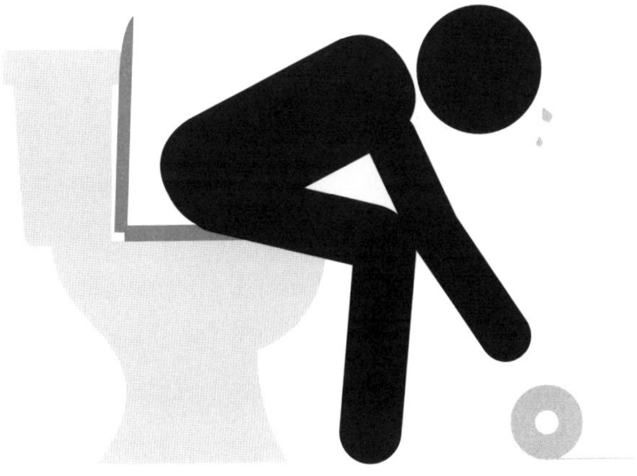

The Downhill

DIFFICULTY RATING:

This is for your inner Olympic skier.
Imagine you're racing down the
mountain, back straight but leaning
forward to go faster, with your arms
behind as far as they will go, like
wings. Now you're soaring!

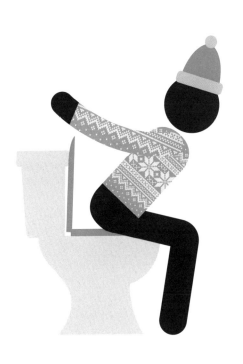

Nose Holds

This one's for after your movements have begun. If they've got a particular whiff to them (much more common if you've been indulging in a particularly protein-rich diet to aid your workouts) then raise your elbow to the height of your ear, reach across your face and hold your nose. As you start to feel the burn (in your arm and hopefully not your nostrils!), switch arms.

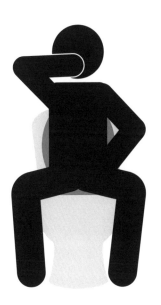

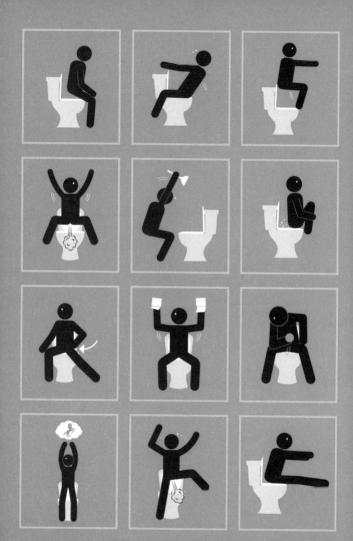

Advanced SHIIT Exercises

This SHIIT just got real. If you've made it this far, then you have bowels of steel, my friend.

The Turtle's Head

DIFFICULTY RATING:

You've pushed a little too much and now there's a turtle's head poking out. It's time to suck it back in! Raise yourself off the seat until you can feel the strain on your knees. Hold position for five and drop back down. Repeat five times.

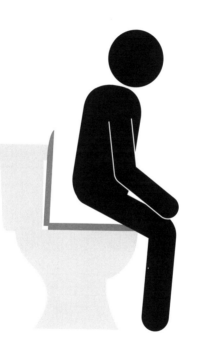

Shit-Ups

DIFFICULTY RATING:

This is only for the well-honed ass-thletes!
Straddle the toilet backwards, gripping
the bowl with your legs. Lower your torso
to a horizontal position and bring it back
up again. An intense workout, so best
attempted after you've worked out the
other thing you came to the toilet for...

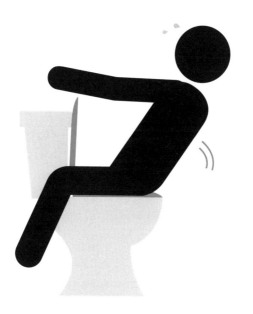

Deep Squat Squit

DIFFICULTY RATING:

It's time to bring on those squits.
Leap onto the seat and squat down
low! Then leap off and squat, then
on and squat. If your eyes aren't
watering, you're not doing it properly!

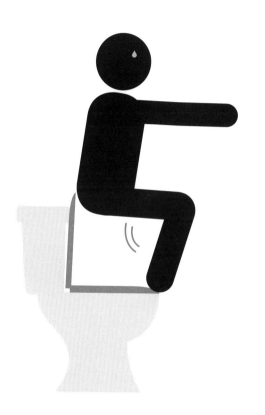

Jumping Jacksies

DIFFICULTY RATING:

Just imagine you've been startled by a giant spider climbing up the wall in front of you. Raise your ass off the seat before jumping into a star shape with your arms and legs wide. This move is particularly effective for dislodging those cling-on plops that don't want to budge. Repeat five times.

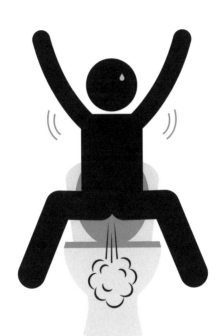

Feel the Force!

DIFFICULTY RATING:

It's time to grab the plunger and show
number two who's boss! Stand facing
the toilet, plunger in your right hand.
Bend over, hinging at the hips and pump
that plunger into the bowl! Complete
five sets, alternating between the left
and right hand. It's a tsunami in there!

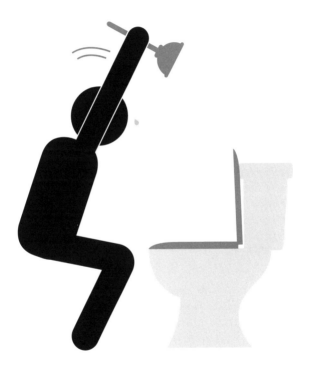

Poo Glitter Bomb

DIFFICULTY RATING:

This is the exercise for those who like to force a trump, leading to poo glitter, which is just like normal glitter but it's not sparkly. Bring in those knees and hold firmly with arms around your calves. Hold for a count of five and release.

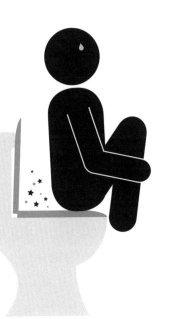

Brown Thunder

DIFFICULTY RATING:

I hear a rumble from deep down below.
There's a storm coming and it won't be
stopped! This one might just shatter the
bowl. Extend one leg out to the side and
pivot in the same direction with your hip,
then draw the leg back in and repeat
on the other side. Do ten sets. Feel
the burn! You're getting SHIIT done!

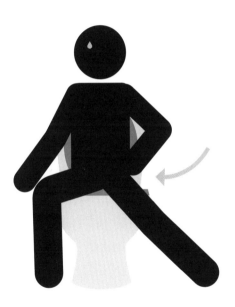

Drop
a Smash

DIFFICULTY RATING:

Grab two toilet rolls, one for each
hand, and lift them above the head,
then behind the head and hold it in
position for a count of five. Repeat
ten times before bringing them to the
front and dropping to the ground.

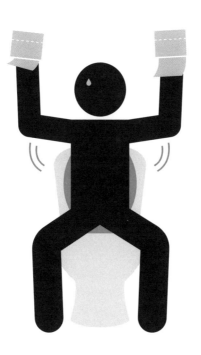

Pan-Jammer Curl

DIFFICULTY RATING:

You'll need a prop for this one; you could use a particularly heavy odour-eating candle or an industrial-sized air freshener. Hold the item in your hand with your arm straight down, and as you curl one out, bend your arm at the elbow.

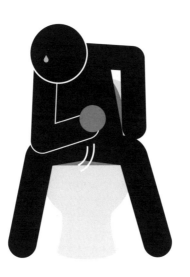

The Poo-nicorn

That rarest of poos, the one that ends in a point. It's almost too perfect to flush away. Salute it by making a point with your arms aloft and your hands together, and rise slowly and majestically from the toilet, keeping knees bent. Hold this position for ten seconds.

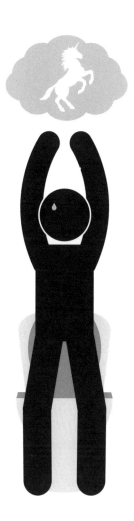

Furious Fartees!

DIFFICULTY RATING:

It's time to increase the pace with some fartees – not to be confused with burpees. Stand up and do a jump. If you're feeling particularly gaseous, extend one leg as you jump. Repeat five times.

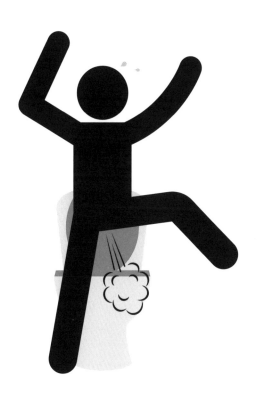

Shartnado

DIFFICULTY RATING:

This is the moment when you can no longer hold in the shitstorm that is about to descend into the toilet. Stretch arms and legs in front of you and hold your position until the dastardly deed is done.

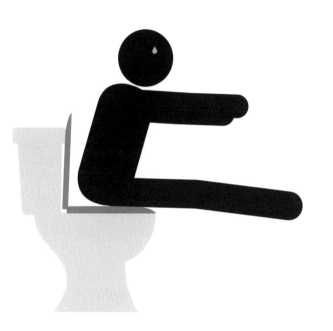

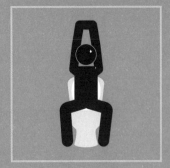
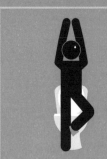
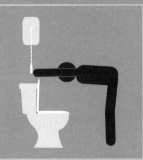
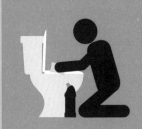
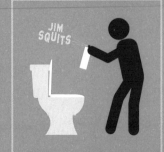

JIM SQUITS

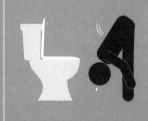

Cool Down

After such a huge physical outlay, it's time to relax those muscles with some cooling down exercises. First, take a minute to reflect on your workout and then enjoy this collection of soothing movements.

Bum
Salutation

DIFFICULTY RATING:

Find relaxation with some light yoga.
Bring your arms straight above
your head with your palms touching
and raise your head to salute
your bum for all its hard work.

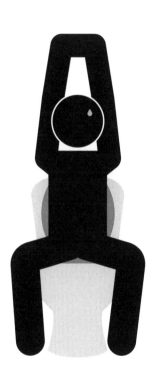

The
Toilet-Tree

DIFFICULTY RATING:

Being able to stand on one leg is a useful
skill in the bathroom, especially when
you get toilet roll stuck to your foot.

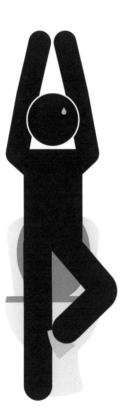

The Power Flush

DIFFICULTY RATING:

Stand up from the toilet and hinge
on the hips, then reach for that chain
and pull like you've never pulled
before. Wave goodbye to your poo
with your free hand (optional).

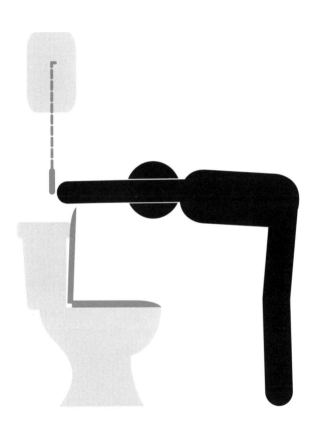

The Safety Wipe

Surely this should be one of the Ten Commandments: Always leave the toilet as you wish to receive it. So, depending on the intensity of your session, get out the cleaning products and scrub that seat in a slow, fluid motion.

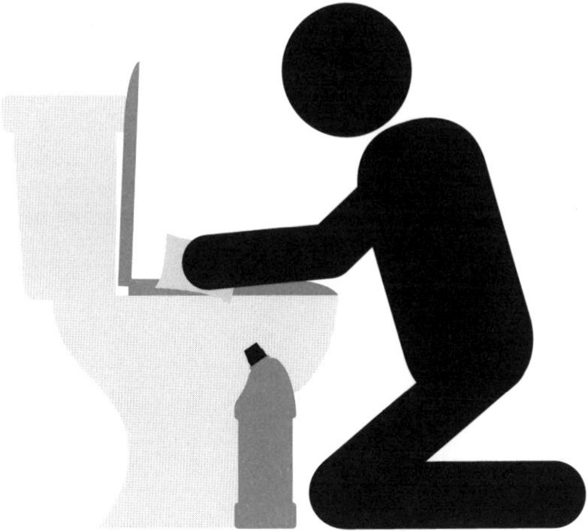

The Neutralizer

DIFFICULTY RATING: 💩

Grab that can of poo-eze and spray as if you're adding a signature to your (f)artful smell. Be proud of what you have achieved today. This is what hard work smells like.

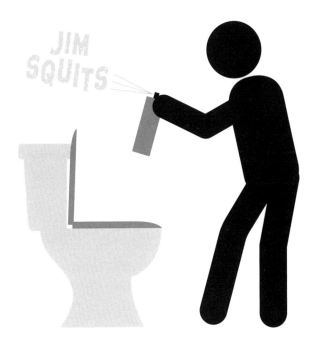

The Ascender

Arise from the porcelain throne
for the last time, then reach down
to the floor, before grabbing your
undercrackers and pulling them up.

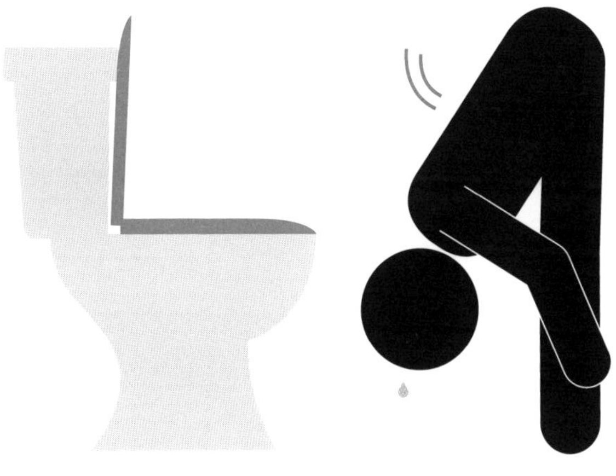

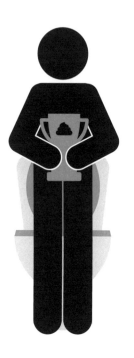

Congratulations

You've strained, you've heaved, you've tooted that butt trumpet, and you've achieved some monster SHIITs. This workout isn't for the meek; it's survival of the SHIITest! Here's your trophy for showing that SHIIT who's boss. Your work is done, my friend. It's time to leave this foul-smelling place for you have stormed that SHIIT workout!

Log Your Workouts

Date	Description	Score out of 10

Date	Description	Score out of 10

Add your own
SHIIT moves

- _____
- _____
- _____
- _____
- _____
- _____
- _____
- _____
- _____
- _____
- _____
- _____
- _____
- _____

Achievement List

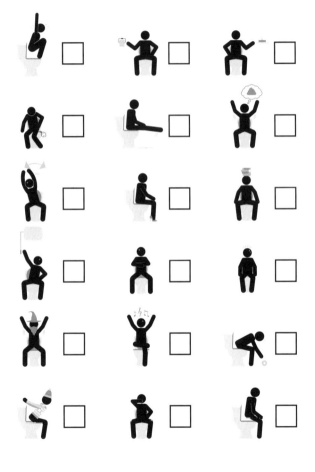

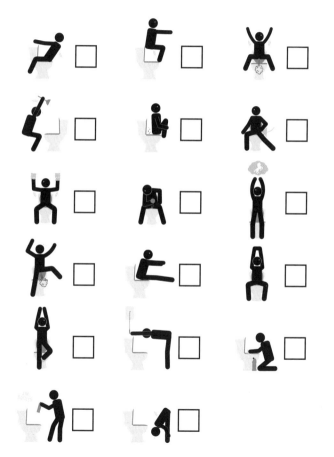

If you're interested in finding out more about our books, find us on Facebook at Summersdale Publishers and follow us on Twitter at @Summersdale.

www.summersdale.com